Special Plant-Based Diet Cooking Guide

A Full Collection of Plant-Based Diet Recipes

Luke Gorman

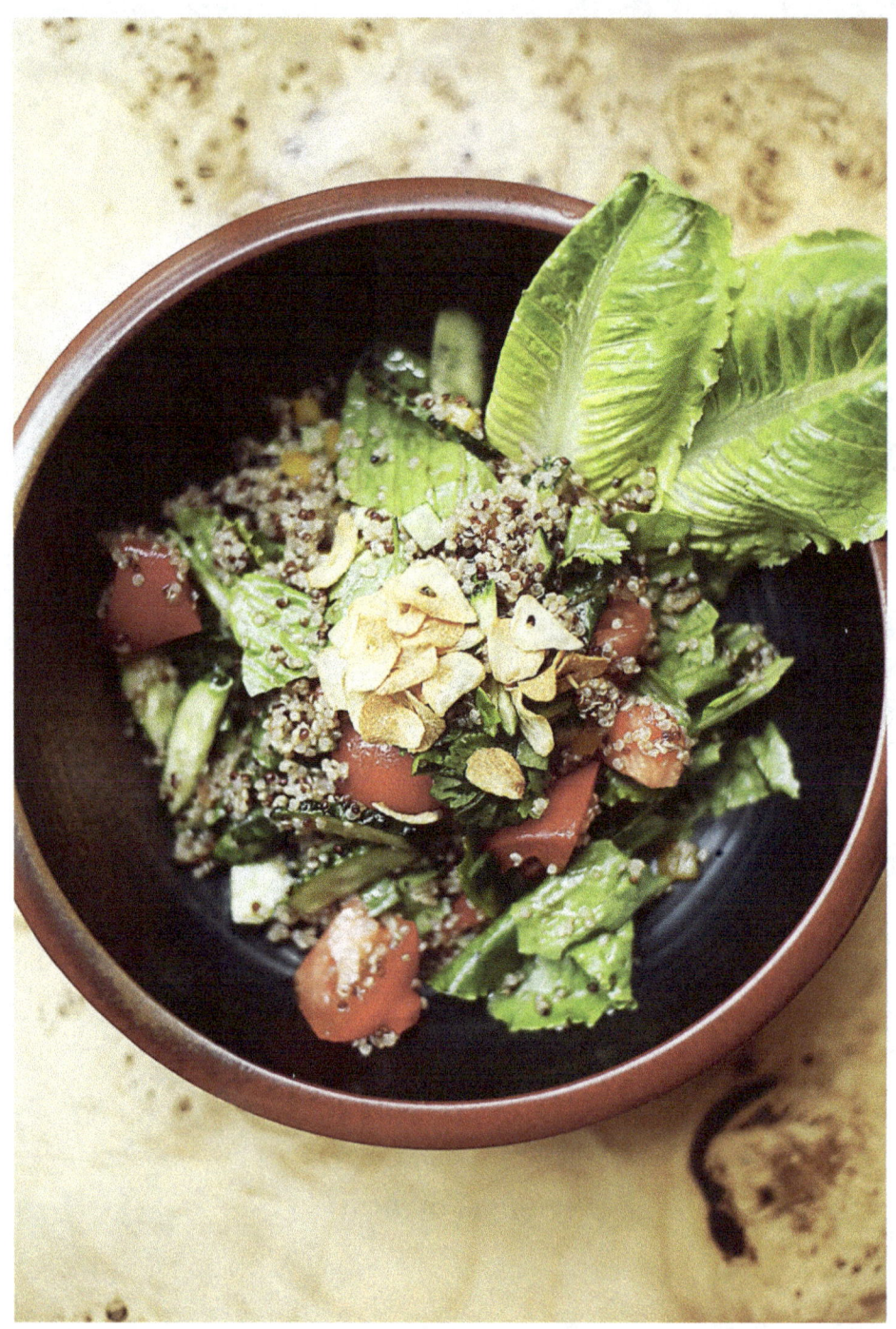

© Copyright 2021 - All rights reserved.

The content contained within this book may not be reproduced, duplicated or transmitted without direct written permission from the author or the publisher.

Under no circumstances will any blame or legal responsibility be held against the publisher, or author, for any damages, reparation, or monetary loss due to the information contained within this book. Either directly or indirectly.

Legal Notice:

This book is copyright protected. This book is only for personal use. You cannot amend, distribute, sell, use, quote or paraphrase any part, or the content within this book, without the consent of the author or publisher.

Disclaimer Notice:

Please note the information contained within this document is for educational and entertainment purposes only. All effort has been executed to present accurate, up to date, and reliable, complete information. No warranties of any kind are declared or implied. Readers acknowledge that the author is not engaging in the rendering of legal, financial, medical or professional advice. The content within this book has been derived from various sources. Please consult a licensed professional before attempting any techniques outlined in this book.

By reading this document, the reader agrees that under no circumstances is the author responsible for any losses, direct or indirect, which are incurred as a result of the use of information contained within this document, including, but not limited to, — errors, omissions, or inaccuracies.

TABLE OF CONTENTS

INTRODUCTION 8

OATMEAL PANCAKE 11

AVOCADO & EGG SALAD ON TOASTED BREAD 14

MOZZARELLA AND CASHEW CHEESE SAUCE 16

EVERYDAY CANTANKEROUS KALE CHIPS 18

TOFU POKE 20

CHILLED TOMATO SOUP 22

BURST YOUR BELLY VEGAN TORTILLA SOUP 25

PROTEIN-REVVING LENTIL VEGETABLE SOUP 28

KIMCHI PASTA 31

GARLIC LEMON MUSHROOMS 33

GRILLED SPICY EGGPLANT 35

ZUCCHINI GARLIC FRIES 37

PROVOLONE OVER HERBED PORTOBELLO MUSHROOMS 39

BLUE CHEESE, FIG AND ARUGULA SALAD 41

PAPRIKA 'N CAJUN SEASONED ONION RINGS 43

VEGETABLE SOUP 45

SPINACH & TOMATO COUSCOUS 48

BASIL RISOTTO 50

WILD RICE SOUP 52

BRUSSELS SPROUT AND LENTIL SOUP 55

GREEN LENTIL SOUP WITH RICE 57

BEAN AND PASTA SOUP 59

SPICED CITRUS BEAN SOUP 62

CURRIED LENTIL SQUASH STEW 64

RICH RED LENTIL CURRY 66

PAPRIKA BROCCOLI 68

CAJUN ONION MIX 70

GREEN BEANS SIDE SALAD 72

WHITE MUSHROOMS MIX 74

MUSHROOMS AND WATERCRESS SALAD 76

LIMA BEAN SALAD 79

EXQUISITE BANANA, APPLE, AND COCONUT CURRY 82

DELIGHTFUL COCONUT VEGETARIAN CURRY 84

CREAMY SWEET POTATO & COCONUT CURRY 86

CHIVES FENNEL SALSA 89

BLUEBERRY, HAZELNUT AND HEMP SMOOTHIE 92

MOCHA CHOCOLATE SHAKE 94

RED BEET, PEAR AND APPLE SMOOTHIE 97

CHOCOLATE AND CHERRY SMOOTHIE 99

BANANA AND PROTEIN SMOOTHIE 101

CONCLUSION 104

Introduction

A plant-based eating routine backing and upgrades the entirety of this. For what reason should most of what we eat originate from the beginning?

Eating more plants is the first nourishing convention known to man to counteract and even turn around the ceaseless diseases that assault our general public.

Plants and vegetables are brimming with large scale and micronutrients that give our bodies all that we require for a sound and productive life. By eating, at any rate, two suppers stuffed with veggies consistently, and nibbling on foods grown from the ground in the middle of, the nature of your wellbeing and at last your life will improve.

The most widely recognized wellbeing worries that individuals have can be reduced by this one straightforward advance.

Things like weight, inadequate rest, awful skin, quickened maturing, irritation, physical torment, and absence of vitality would all be able to be decidedly influenced by expanding the admission of plants and characteristic nourishments.

If you're reading this book, then you're probably on a journey to get healthy because you know good health and nutrition go hand in hand.

Maybe you're looking at the plant-based diet as a solution to those love handles.

Whatever the case may be, the standard American diet millions of people eat daily is not the best way to fuel your body.

If you ask me, any other diet will already be a significant improvement. Since what you eat fuels your body, you can imagine that eating junk will make you feel just that—like junk.

I've followed the standard American diet for several years: my plate was loaded with high-fat and carbohydrate-rich foods. I know this doesn't sound like a horrible way to eat, but keep in mind that most Americans don't focus on eating healthy fats and complex carbs—we live on processed foods.

The consequences of eating foods filled with trans fats, preservatives, and mountains of sugar are fatigue, reduced mental focus, mood swings, and weight gain. To top it off, there's the issue of opening yourself up to certain diseases—some life-threatening—when you neglect paying attention to what you eat .

Oatmeal Pancake

Preparation Time: 10 minutes

Cooking Time: 30 minutes

Servings: 8

Ingredients:

- ½ cup blueberries
- 3 bananas, sliced
- 2 tsp. lemon juice
- ¼ cup maple syrup
- ¼ tsp. ground cinnamon
- 1 cup flour
- 2 tsp. baking powder
- ½ tsp. baking soda
- ½ cup rolled oats
- Salt to taste

- 1 egg, beaten
- 1 cup buttermilk
- 1 tsp. vanilla
- 1 tbsp. olive oil

Directions:

1. Toss the blueberries and bananas in lemon juice, maple syrup and cinnamon.
2. Set aside.
3. In a bowl, mix the flour, baking powder, baking soda, oats and salt.
4. In another bowl, combine the egg, milk and vanilla.
5. Slowly add the second bowl mixture into the first one.
6. Mix well.
7. Pour the oil into a pan over medium heat.
8. Pour 4 tablespoons of the batter and cook for 2 minutes per side.
9. Repeat with the remaining batter.
10. Serve the pancakes with the fruits.

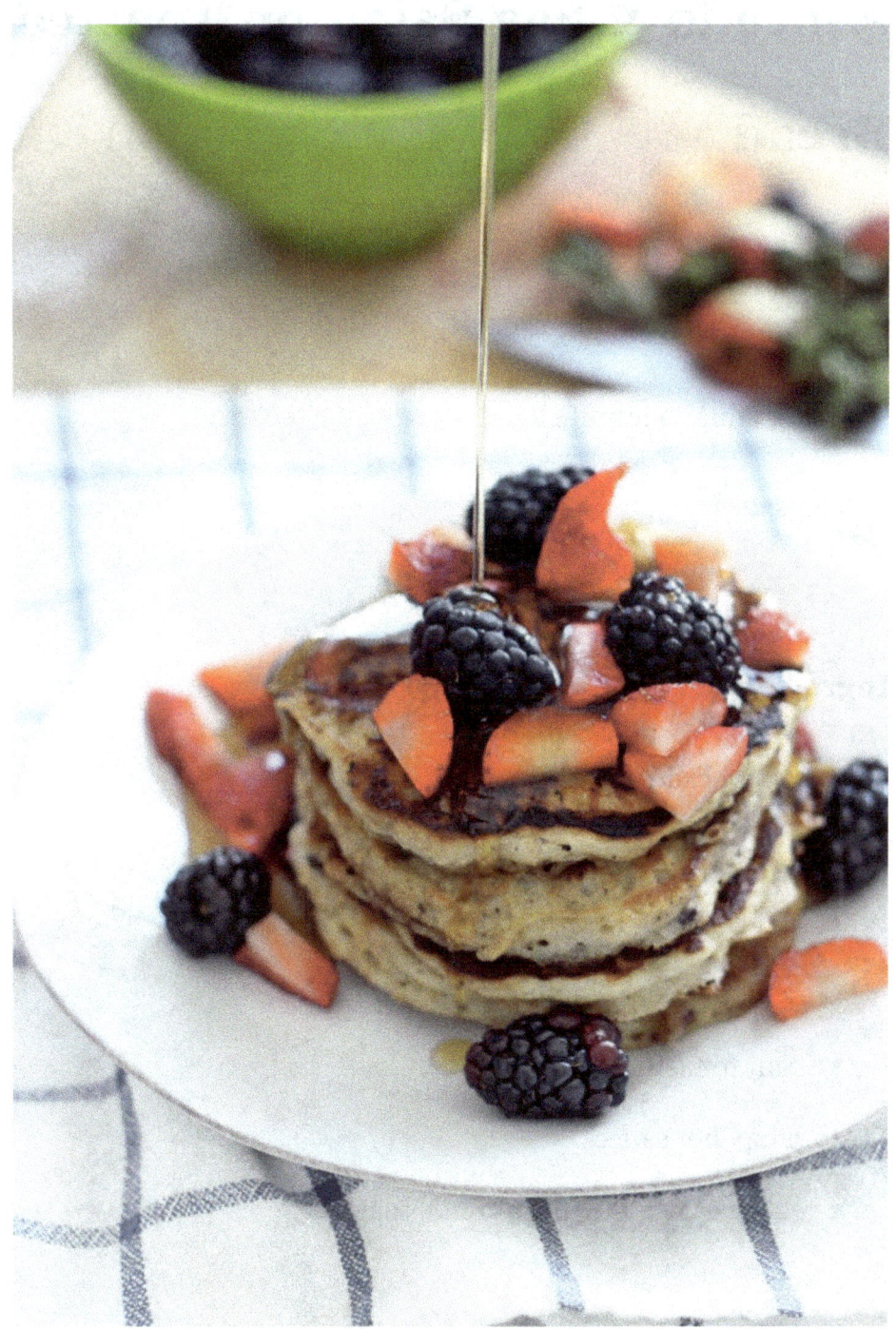

Avocado & Egg Salad on Toasted Bread

Preparation Time: 5 minutes

Cooking Time: 0 minute

Servings: 2

Ingredients:

- ½ avocado
- 1 tsp. lemon juice
- 2 hard-boiled egg, chopped
- 2 tbsp. celery, chopped
- Salt to taste
- 1 tsp. hot sauce
- 2 slices whole-wheat bread, toasted

Directions:

1. Mash the avocado in a bowl.
2. Stir in the lemon juice, egg, celery, salt and hot sauce.
3. Spread the mixture on top of the toasted bread.

Mozzarella and Cashew Cheese Sauce

Preparation Time: 20minutes

Ingredients:

- 1 cup of water
- 2 tablespoons lemon juice
- 2 tablespoons cornstarch

Directions:

1. Soak the cashews for at least 4 hours or overnight.
2. Put all the INGREDIENTS in the blender and stir until smooth.
3. Pour over pizza or nachos and bake.

4. The cornstarch makes the sauce slightly firm when baked and creates a beautifully baked crust.
5. It lasts only about three days in the fridge, but can be kept in the freezer for about a month.
6. You just need to be completely defrosted before using it.

Everyday Cantankerous Kale Chips

Preparation time: 10 minutes

Cooking time: 25 minutes

Servings: 6.

Ingredients:

- 12 ounces kale
- 1 tbsp. olive oil
- salt to taste

Directions:

1. Begin by de-stemming the kale and tearing the kale into chip-like pieces.
2. Rinse these leaves, and allow them to dry completely.

3. After they've dried, preheat the oven to 325 degrees Fahrenheit.
4. Next, place the kale in a mixing bowl, and drizzle about a tbsp. of olive oil overtop of them.
5. Mix up the kale to coat it with the oil.
6. Place the kale leaves out on a baking sheet in one layer, and bake the kale chips for twenty minutes.
7. After you remove the kale leaves, salt them and enjoy!

Tofu Poke

Serves: 4

Time: 30 Minutes

Ingredients:

- ¾ Cup Scallions, Sliced Thin
- 1 ½ Tablespoons Mirin
- ¼ Cup Tamari
- 1 ½ Tablespoon Dark Sesame Oil, Toasted
- 1 Tablespoon Sesame Seeds, Toasted (Optional)
- 2 Teaspoons Ginger, fresh & Grated
- ½ Teaspoon Red Pepper, crushed
- 12 Ounces Extra Firm Tofu, Drained & Cut into ½ Inch Pieces
- 4 Cups Zucchini Noodles
- 2 Tablespoons Rice Vinegar

- 2 Cups Carrots, Shredded
- 2 Cups Pea Shoots
- ¼ Cup Basil, Fresh & Chopped
- ¼ Cup Peanuts, Toasted & Chopped (Optional)

Directions:

1. Wisk your tamari, mirin, sesame seeds, oil, ginger, red pepper, and scallion greens in a bowl.
2. Set two tablespoons of this sauce aside, and add the tofu to the remaining sauce.
3. Toss to coat.
4. Combine your vinegar and zucchini noodles in a bowl.
5. Divide it between four bowls, topping with tofu, carrots, and a tablespoon of basil and peanuts.
6. Drizzle with sauce before serving.

Chilled Tomato Soup

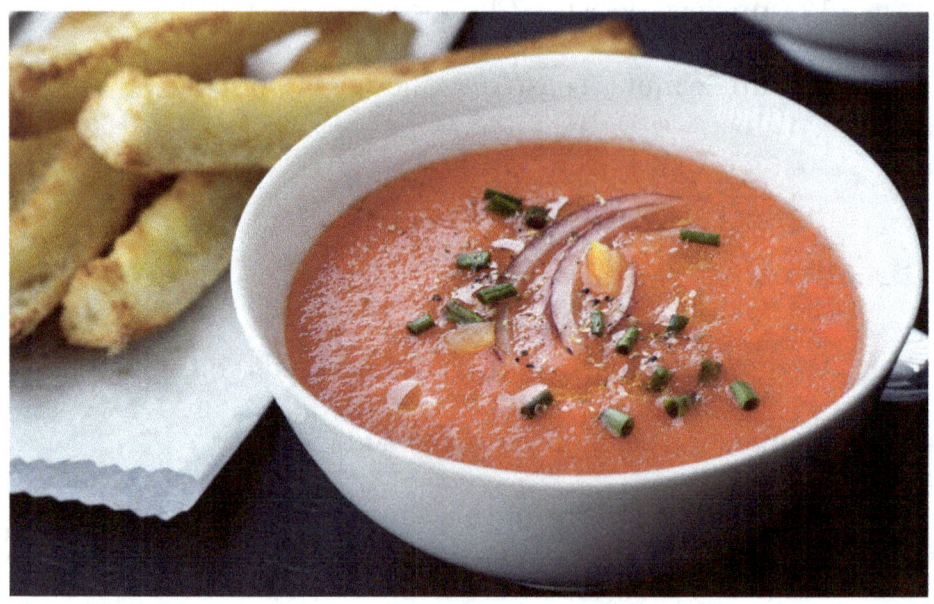

Preparation time: 5 minutes

Cooking time: 50 minutes

Servings: 3

Ingredients:

- 6 tomatoes, medium-sized
- 1 cucumber, chopped
- ½ cup onion, chopped finely
- 4 tsp. lemon juice
- 1 Tbs. lemon rind, grated
- 1 cup sour cream
- ½ tsp. ginger
- 1 large cantaloupe
- 1 Tbs. dried basil, crushed
- 2½ tsp. salt pepper to taste

Directions:

1. Put the tomatoes in boiling water for a few minutes, until the skins start to crack and peel.
2. Remove the tomatoes and peel them.
3. Purée them in a blender or food processor at high speed.
4. You should have 5 cups of the fresh tomato purée.
5. Purée the cucumber and onions in a blender or food processor and add this to the tomatoes.

6. If you are using a blender, you could "prime" it with a bit of the puréed tomatoes.
7. Stir in the sour cream and season the soup with salt, ginger, pepper, lemon juice, and lemon rind.
8. Halve the cantaloupe, remove all the seeds, and either cut it into small balls with a melon scoop or peel and cut it into chunks.
9. Toss the melon with the chopped basil and chill both soup and melon for several hours.
10. To serve, pour the soup into chilled bowls and put a few spoonful of the melon into each one.

Burst Your Belly Vegan Tortilla Soup

Preparation time: 5 minutes

Cooking time: 40 minutes

6 Servings.

Ingredients:

- 3 minced garlic cloves
- 1 tbsp. olive oil
- 1 diced onion
- ¾ cup quinoa
- 1 diced green pepper
- 32 ounces vegetable broth
- 1 diced zucchini
- 6 corn tortillas

- 1 16 ounce can of diced tomatoes
- 1 tsp. cumin
- ½ tsp. oregano salt and pepper to taste

Directions:

1. Begin by heating the oil in a soup pan, and adding the garlic and the onion to the oil.
2. Cook these for five minutes.
3. Afterwards, add the quinoa, the broth, and the bell pepper.
4. Bring this mixture to a boil.
5. Afterwards, lower the heat and allow it to simmer for fifteen minutes.
6. Next, slice up the tortillas into small strips and heat them in a skillet with a little olive oil in order to toast them.
7. Now, add the zucchini, the cumin, and the oregano to the soup.
8. Stir, and allow it to simmer for fifteen more minutes.

9. Add salt and pepper, and serve warm with tortilla strips overtop.

10. Enjoy!

Protein-Revving Lentil Vegetable Soup

Preparation time: 5 minutes

Cooking time: 50 minutes

8 Servings.

Ingredients:

- 3 minced garlic cloves
- 1 diced onion
- 3 tbsp. olive oil
- 2 sliced carrots
- 2 diced celery stalks
- 5 cups water
- 2 diced potatoes
- 1 tbsp. Italian herbs

- 1 ½ cups green lentils
- 2 tsp. paprika
- 16 ounces diced tomatoes
- 1/3 cup chopped cilantro

Directions:

1. Begin by heating the oil and the vegetables together in the bottom of a soup pot.
2. Saute the vegetables for about ten minutes.
3. Afterwards, add the water, the lentils, the potatoes, the seasoning, and the paprika.
4. Stir, and allow the mixture to simmer for thirty minutes with the cover on.
5. Next, place the cilantro in the soup and allow it to simmer for twenty more minutes.
6. Serve with a bit of salt and pepper, and enjoy.

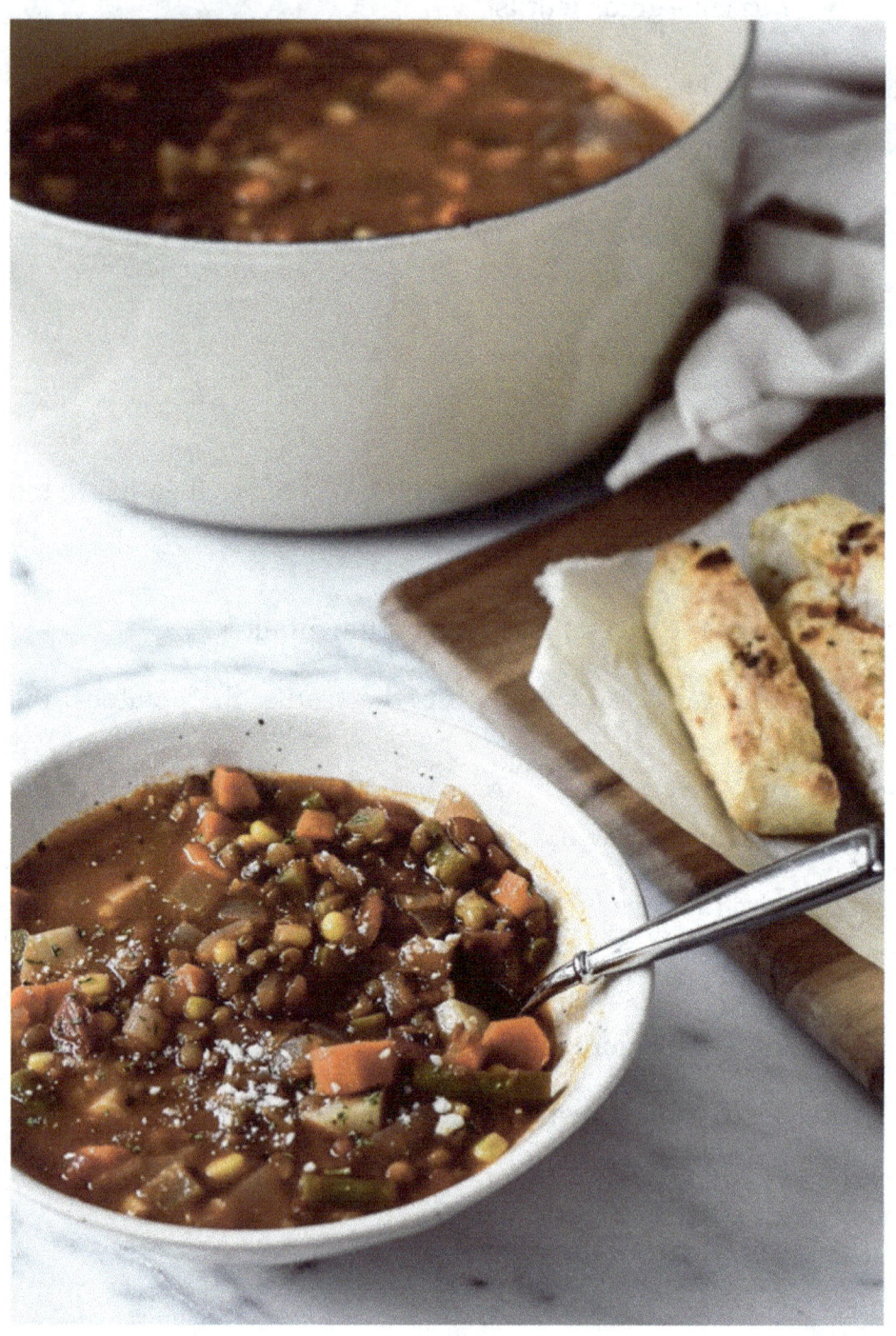

Kimchi Pasta

Preparation time: 5 minutes

Cooking time: 25 minutes

Servings: 4

Ingredients:

- 2 1/3 Cup Vegetable Stock
- 8 Ounces Small Pasta
- 2 Cloves Garlic, Minced
- ½ Red Onion, Sliced
- 1 Teaspoon Sea Salt, Fine
- 1 ¼ Cups Kimchi, Chopped
- ½ Cup Cashew Sour Cream

Directions:

1. Combine the stock, garlic, red onion, pasta and salt in your instant pot.
2. Lock the lid, and cook on high pressure for a minute.
3. Use a quick release, and then press sauté and set it to low.
4. Stir the kimchi in, and allow it to simmer for three minutes.
5. Stir in the sour cream before serving warm.

Garlic Lemon Mushrooms

Preparation time: 15 minutes

Cooking time: 20 minutes

Servings: 4

Ingredients:

- 1/4 cup lemon juice
- 3 tablespoons minced fresh parsley
- 3 garlic cloves, minced
- 1-pound large fresh mushrooms

What you'll need from the store cupboard:

- Pepper to taste
- 4 tablespoons olive oil

Directions

1. For the dressing, whisk together the first 5 ingredients.
2. Toss mushrooms with 2 tablespoons dressing.
3. Grill mushrooms, covered, over medium-high heat until tender, 5-7 minutes per side.
4. Toss with remaining dressing before serving.

Grilled Spicy Eggplant

Preparation time: 20 minutes

Cooking time: 20 minutes

Servings: 2

Ingredients:

- 2 small eggplants, cut into 1/2-inch slices
- 1/4 cup olive oil
- 2 tablespoons lime juice
- 3 teaspoons Cajun seasoning

What you'll need from the store cupboard:

- Salt and pepper to taste

Directions:

1. Brush eggplant slices with oil.

2. Drizzle with lime juice; sprinkle with Cajun seasoning.

3. Let stand for 5 minutes.

4. Grill eggplant, covered, over medium heat or broil 4 minutes.

5. From heat until tender, 4-5 minutes per side.

6. Season with pepper and salt to taste. Serve and enjoy.

Zucchini Garlic Fries

Preparation time: minutes

Cooking time: 25 minutes

Servings: 6

Ingredients:

- ¼ teaspoon garlic powder
- ½ cup almond flour
- 2 large egg, beaten
- 3 medium zucchinis, sliced into fry sticks
- 3 tablespoons olive oil

What you'll need from the store cupboard:

- Salt and pepper to taste

Directions

1. Preheat oven to 400oF.
2. Mix all ingredients in a bowl until the zucchini fries are well coated.
3. Place fries on a cookie sheet and spread evenly.
4. Put in the oven and cook for 15 minutes.
5. Stir fries, continue baking for an additional 10 minutes.

Provolone Over Herbed Portobello Mushrooms

Preparation time: 10 minutes

Cooking time: 10 minutes

Servings: 2

Ingredients:

- 2 Portobello mushrooms, stemmed and wiped clean
- 1 tsp minced garlic
- ¼ tsp dried rosemary
- 1 tablespoon balsamic vinegar
- ¼ cup grated provolone cheese

What you'll need from the store cupboard:

- 4 tablespoons olive oil
- Salt and pepper to taste

Directions

1. In an oven, position rack 4-inches away from the top and preheat broiler.
2. Prepare a baking dish by spraying with cooking spray lightly.
3. Stemless, place mushroom gill side up.
4. Mix well garlic, rosemary, balsamic vinegar, and olive oil in a small bowl.
5. Season with salt and pepper to taste.
6. Drizzle over mushrooms equally.
7. Marinate for at least 5 minutes before popping into the oven and broiling for 4 minutes per side or until tender.
8. Once cooked, remove from oven, sprinkle cheese, return to broiler and broil for a minute or two or until cheese melts.
9. Remove from oven and serve right away.

Blue Cheese, Fig and Arugula Salad

Preparation time: 10 minutes

Cooking time: 0 minutes

Servings: 4

Ingredients:

- 1 tsp Dijon mustard
- 3 tbsp Balsamic Vinegar
- ¼ cup crumbled blue cheese
- 2 bags arugula
- 1 fig fruit, sliced
- ½ cup walnuts, chopped

What you'll need from the store cupboard:

- Pepper and salt to taste

- 5 tbsp olive oil

Directions

1. Whisk thoroughly together pepper, salt, olive oil, Dijon mustard, and balsamic vinegar to make the dressing.
2. Set aside in the ref for at least 30 minutes to marinate and allow the spices to combine.
3. On four serving plates, evenly arrange arugula and top with blue cheese, figs, and walnuts
4. Drizzle each plate of salad with 1 ½ tbsp of prepared dressing.
5. Serve and enjoy.

Paprika 'n Cajun Seasoned Onion Rings

Preparation time: 15 minutes

Cooking time: 25 minutes

Servings: 6

Ingredients:

- 1 large white onion
- 2 large eggs, beaten
- ½ teaspoon Cajun seasoning
- ¾ cup almond flour
- 1 ½ teaspoon paprika

What you'll need from the store cupboard:

- ½ cups coconut oil for frying
- ¼ cup water

- Salt and pepper to taste

Directions

1. Preheat a pot with oil for 8 minutes.
2. Peel the onion, cut off the top and slice into circles.
3. In a mixing bowl, combine the water and the eggs.
4. Season with pepper and salt.
5. Soak the onion in the egg mixture.
6. In another bowl, combine the almond flour, paprika powder, Cajun seasoning, salt and pepper.
7. Dredge the onion in the almond flour mixture.
8. Place in the pot and cook in batches until golden brown, around 8 minutes per batch.

Vegetable Soup

Preparation time: 5 minutes

Cooking time: 40 minutes

Servings: 6

Ingredients:

- 12 Ounces Green Beans
- 1 Can Tomatoes, Diced
- 1 Onion, Chopped
- 12 Ounces Mixed Vegetables, Frozen
- 2 ¾ Cup Vegetable Broth

Directions:

1. Press sauté, and then add in some cooking oil.
2. Add the onion, and sauté for two minutes.

3. Stir in the remaining ingredients.
4. Seal the lid, and then cook on high pressure for five minutes.
5. Use a natural release for five minutes before finishing with a quick release.
6. Serve warm.

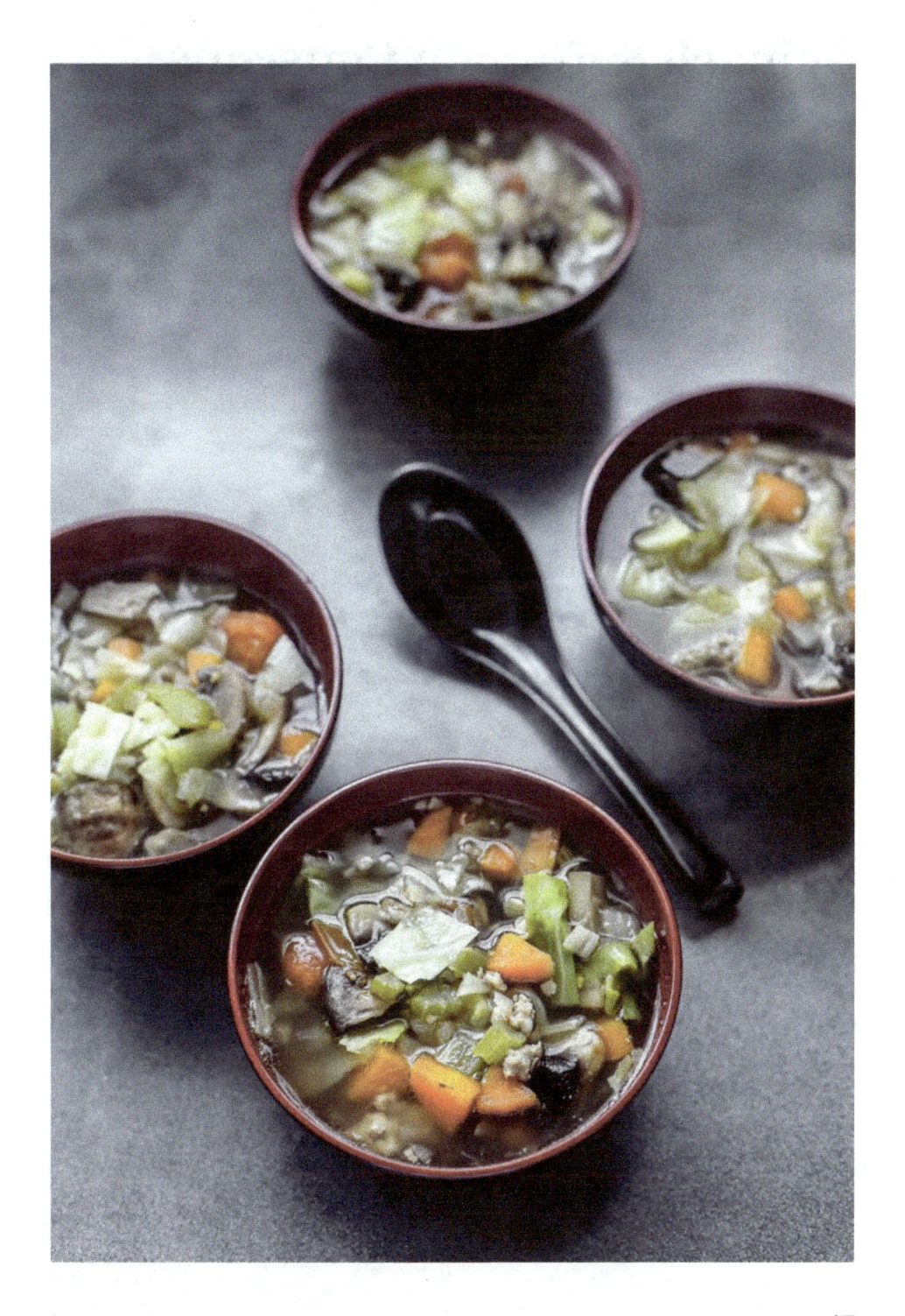

Spinach & Tomato Couscous

Preparation time: 5 minutes

Cooking time: 35 minutes

Servings: 4

Ingredients:

- 1 ¼ Vegetable Broth
- 8 Ounces Couscous
- 1 ½ Cups Tomatoes, Chopped
- 2 Tablespoons Vegan Butter
- ½ Cup Spinach, Fresh & Chopped

Directions:

1. Press sauté on your instant pot, and melt your butter.

2. Once the butter I smelted, stir in the couscous, allowing it to cook for a minute.
3. Pour in the broth, and stir well before sealing the lid.
4. Cook on high pressure for five minutes, and then use a quick release.
5. Stir in your tomato and spinach, and serve warm.

Basil Risotto

Preparation time: 5 minutes

Cooking time: 40 minutes

Servings: 6

Ingredients:

- 1 Onion, Chopped
- 1 ½ Tablespoons Olive Oil
- 28 Ounces Vegetable Broth
- 12 Ounces Arborio Rice
- 1 ½ Cups Basil, Chopped & Fresh

Directions:

1. Turn your instant pot on sauté and warm your oil.
2. Chop the onions before adding them.

3. Cook for three minutes, and then add in your rice.
4. Cook for a minute more before adding in your broth.
5. Stir well, and then seal the lid.
6. Cook for fifteen minutes on high pressure.
7. Use a quick release, and then press sauté.
8. Cook for one more minute, and then serve warm.

Wild Rice Soup

Preparation time: 5 minutes

Cooking time: 20 minutes

Servings: 4

Ingredients:

- 8 Ounces Baby Bella Mushrooms, Sliced
- 2 Bay leaves
- ½ Teaspoon Thyme
- ½ Teaspoon Paprika
- 4 Cloves Garlic, Minced
- 1 Sweet Onion, Small & Diced
- 5 Carrots, Sliced
- 5 Celery Stalks, Sliced
- 8 Tablespoons Vegan Butter, Divided
- ½ Teaspoon Sea Salt

- 4 Cups Vegetable Stock
- ½ Cups All Purpose Flour
- 1 Cup Coconut Milk
- 1 Cup Wild Rice
- Black Pepper to Taste

Directions:

1. Press sauté, and then add in your butter.
2. Once your butter has melted, add in your celery, carrots, onion, mushrooms, garlic, paprika, bay leaves, thyme and salt.
3. Cook for three minutes, and then turn it off of sauté.
4. Stir in the wild rice and stock.
5. Seal the lid, and then cook on high pressure for thirty-five minutes.
6. Get out a small pan and place it over medium-low heat, and then melt six tablespoons of butter.
7. Whisk in your flour, allowing it to cook for four minutes.
8. Whisk in the milk, and make sure to continue whisking until it creates a lump free mixture.

9. Use a quick release, and the discard the bay leaves.
10. Press sauté, and then stir in your butter mixture.
11. Cook until it thickens, and then season with salt and pepper before serving warm.

Brussels Sprout and Lentil Soup

Preparation time: 5 minutes

Cooking time: 40 minutes

Servings: 4

Ingredients:

- 1 cup brown lentils
- 1 onion, chopped
- 2-3 cloves garlic, peeled
- 2 medium carrots, chopped
- 16 oz Brussels sprouts, shredded
- 4 cups vegetable broth
- 4 tbsp olive oil
- 1 ½ tsp paprika
- 1 tsp summer savory

Directions:

1. Heat oil in a deep soup pot, add the onion and carrots and sauté until golden.
2. Add in paprika and lentils with vegetable broth.
3. Bring to the boil, lower heat and simmer for 15-20 minutes.
4. Add the Brussels sprouts and the tomato to the soup, together with the garlic and summer savory.
5. Cook for 15 more minutes, add salt to taste and serve.

Green Lentil Soup with Rice

Preparation time: 5 minutes

Cooking time: 40 minutes

Servings: 6

Ingredients:

- 1 cup green lentils
- 1 small onion, finely cut
- 1 carrot, chopped
- 5 cups vegetable broth
- 1/4 cup rice
- 1 tbsp paprika
- salt and black pepper, to taste
- 1/2 cup finely cut dill, to serve

Directions:

1. Heat oil in a large saucepan and sauté the onion stirring occasionally, until transparent.
2. Add in carrot, paprika and lentils and stir to combine.
3. Add vegetable broth to the saucepan and bring to the boil, then reduce heat and simmer for 20 minutes.
4. Stir in rice and cook on medium low until rice is cooked.
5. Sprinkle with dill and serve.

Bean and Pasta Soup

Preparation time: 5 minutes

Cooking time: 20 minutes

Servings: 6-7

Ingredients:

- 1 cup small pasta, cooked
- 1 cup canned white beans, rinsed and drained
- 2 medium carrots, cut
- 1 cup fresh spinach, torn
- 1 medium onion, chopped
- 1 celery rib, chopped
- 2 garlic cloves, crushed
- 3 cups water
- 1 cup canned tomatoes, diced and undrained
- 1 cup vegetable broth

- ½ tsp rosemary
- ½ tsp basil salt and pepper, to taste

Directions:

1. Add all ingredients except pasta and spinach into slow cooker.
2. Cover and cook on low for 6-7 hours or high for 4 hours.
3. Add spinach and pasta about 30 minutes before the soup is finished cooking.

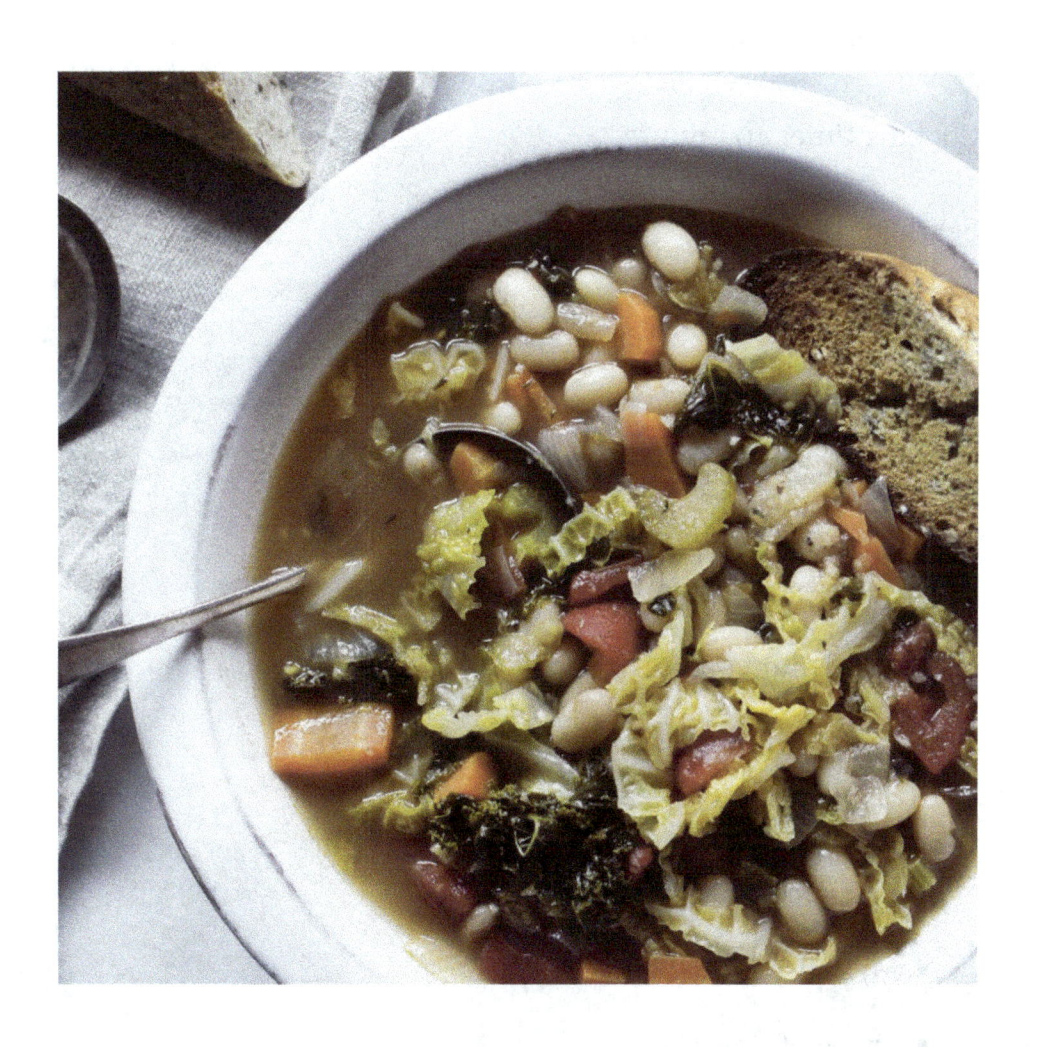

Spiced Citrus Bean Soup

Preparation time: 5 minutes

Cooking time: 40 minutes

Servings: 6-7

Ingredients:

- 1 can (14 oz) white beans, rinsed and drained
- 2 medium carrots, cut
- 1 medium onion, chopped
- 1 tbsp gram masala
- 4 cups vegetable broth
- 1 cup coconut milk
- 1/2 tbsp grated ginger
- juice of 1 orange
- salt and pepper, to taste
- 1/2 cup fresh parsley leaves, finely cut, to serve

Directions:

1. In a large soup pot, sauté onions, carrots and ginger in olive oil, for about 5 minutes, stirring.
2. Add gram masala and cook until just fragrant.
3. Add the orange juice and vegetable broth and bring to the boil.
4. Simmer for about 10 min until the carrots are tender, then stir in the coconut milk.
5. Blend soup to desired consistency then add the beans and bring to a simmer.
6. Serve sprinkled with parsley.

Curried Lentil Squash Stew

Preparation time: 5 minutes

Cooking time: 30 minutes

4 Servings.

Ingredients:

- 1 diced onion
- 1 tsp. olive oil
- 4 minced garlic cloves
- 4 cups vegetable broth
- 1 tbsp. curry powder
- 1 cup red lentils
- 4 cups pre-baked butternut squash
- 1 cup broccoli

Directions:

1. Begin by bringing the oil, the onion, and the garlic together in the bottom of a soup pot for five minutes on medium.
2. Next, add the curry powder, and stir the ingredients for a few minutes.
3. Add the broth and the lentils to the pot, and allow the mixture to simmer for ten minutes.
4. Next, add the pre-baked butternut squash and the broccoli to the mixture.
5. Allow the soup to cook for ten minutes, stirring occasionally.
6. Add salt, pepper, and curry powder to the mixture to your desired taste, and enjoy.

Rich Red Lentil Curry

Servings: 16

Preparation time: 8 hours and 10 minutes

Ingredients:

- 4 cups of brown lentils, uncooked and rinsed
- 2 medium-sized white onions, peeled and diced
- 2 teaspoons of minced garlic
- 1 tablespoon of minced ginger
- 1 teaspoon of salt
- 1/4 teaspoon of cayenne pepper
- 5 tablespoons of red curry paste
- 2 teaspoon of brown sugar
- 1 1/2 teaspoon of ground turmeric
- 1 tablespoon of garam masala
- 60-ounce of tomato puree

- 7 cups of water
- 1/2 cup of coconut milk
- 1/4 cup of chopped cilantro

Directions:

1. Using a 6-quarts slow cooker, place all the ingredients except for the coconut milk and cilantro.
2. Stir until it mixes properly and cover the top.
3. Plug in the slow cooker; adjust the cooking time to 5 hours and let it cook on the high heat setting or until the lentils are soft.
4. Check the curry during cooking and add more water if needed.
5. When the curry is cooked, stir in the milk, then garnish it with the cilantro and serve right away.

Paprika Broccoli

Preparation Time: 10 minutes

Cooking Time: 20 minutes

Servings:

Ingredients

- 1 broccoli head, florets separated
- Juice of ½ lemon
- 1 tablespoon olive oil
- 2 teaspoons paprika
- Salt and black pepper to the taste
- 3 garlic cloves, minced
- 1 tablespoon sesame seeds

Directions:

1. In a bowl, mix broccoli with lemon juice, oil, paprika, salt, pepper and garlic and toss to coat.
2. Transfer to your Air Fryer's basket, cook at 360 ° F for 15 minutes, sprinkle sesame seeds, cook for 5 minutes more, divide between plates and serve as a side dish.

Cajun Onion Mix

Preparation Time: 2 hours

Cooking Time: 15 minutes

Servings:

Ingredients

- 2 big white onions, cut into medium chunks
- Salt and black pepper to the taste
- ¼ cup coconut cream
- A drizzle of olive oil
- 1½ teaspoon paprika
- 1 teaspoon garlic powder
- ½ teaspoon Cajun seasoning

Directions:

1. In a pan that fits your Air Fryer, combine onion chunks with salt, pepper, cream, oil, paprika, garlic powder and Cajun seasoning, toss, introduce the pan in your Air Fryer and cook at 360 ° F for 15 minutes.
2. Divide the onion mix between plates and serve as a side dish.

Green Beans Side Salad

Preparation Time: 10 minutes

Cooking Time: 15 minutes

Servings:

Ingredients

- 1-pint cherry tomatoes
- 1 pound green beans
- 2 tablespoons olive oil
- Salt and black pepper to the taste

Directions:

1. In a bowl, mix cherry tomatoes with green beans, olive oil, salt and pepper, toss, and transfer to a pan that fits your Air Fryer and cook at 400 ° F for 15 minutes.
2. Divide between plates and serve as a side dish.

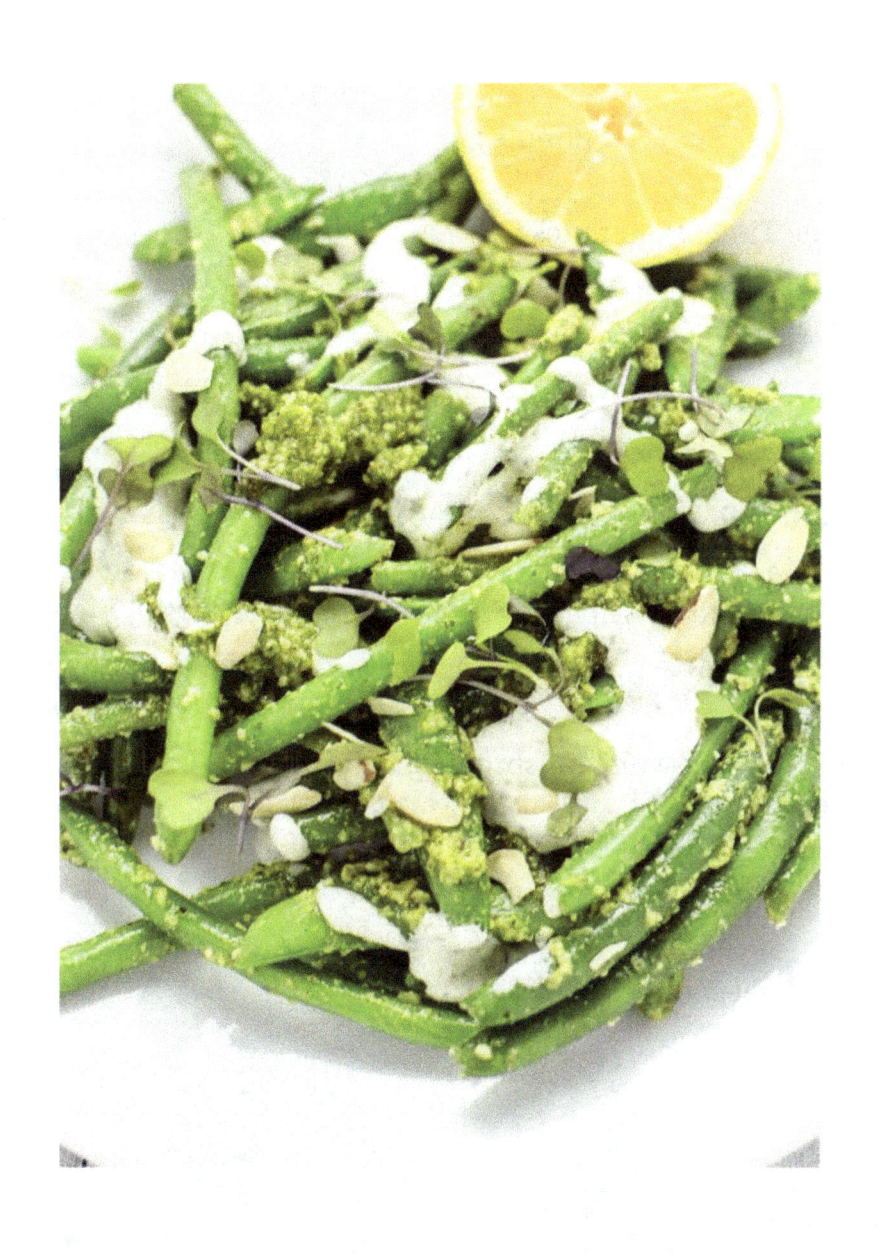

White Mushrooms Mix

Preparation Time: 10 minutes

Cooking Time: 15 minutes

Servings:

Ingredients

- Salt and black pepper to the taste
- 7 ounces snow peas
- 8 ounces white mushrooms, halved
- 1 yellow onion, cut into rings
- 2 tablespoons coconut aminos
- 1 teaspoon olive oil

Directions:

1. In a bowl, snow peas with mushrooms, onion, aminos, oil, salt and pepper, toss well, transfer to a pan that fits your Air Fryer, introduce in the fryer and cook at 350 °F for 15 minutes.
2. Divide between plates and serve as a side dish

Mushrooms and Watercress Salad

Preparation time: 10 minutes

Cooking time: 30 minutes

Servings: 3

Ingredients:

- 8 firm mushrooms, sliced
- 4 eggs, hard-boiled
- 1 bunch watercress
- 1 potato
- ½ medium-sized red onion
- 1 lb. string beans
- 1 medium-small cucumber
- ¾ cup Sour Cream Dressing

- ½ cup mayonnaise

Directions:

1. Peel and dice the potato, cook it in boiling salted water until it is tender, drain, and run cold water over it until it is cool.
2. Put it in the refrigerator.
3. Wash and trim the string beans, cut them in 1-inch pieces, and boil them in salted water until they are just tender—not a minute longer.
4. Run cold water over them until they are cool and put them in the refrigerator.
5. Wash the watercress, trim off the heavy stems, and cut in half any very large pieces.
6. Quarter and thinly slice the red onion.
7. Peel and coarsely chop the hard-boiled eggs.
8. Peel the cucumber, halve it lengthwise, and slice it.
9. Clean the mushrooms, trim off the stems, and slice them thinly.

10. Toss all the vegetable ingredients together in a bowl.

11. Blend Sour Cream Dressing I with the mayonnaise; pour the dressing over the salad and toss again until everything is evenly coated.

Lima Bean Salad

Preparation time: 10 minutes

Cooking time: 40 minutes

Servings: 3

Ingredients:

- 2 cups dry lima beans, large
- ⅓ cup olive oil
- 1½ qts. water
- ¼ cup white wine vinegar
- salt
- fresh-ground black pepper

Directions:

1. Put the beans in a large pot with the water and 1 teaspoon salt, bring to a boil, then reduce the flame.
2. Simmer the beans gently for about 1 hour, or until they are just tender.
3. Drain them while they are still hot, reserving the liquid.
4. In a skillet, boil the bean liquid vigorously for a few minutes until it is substantially thickened.
5. Measure out ⅔ cup of the thickened liquid into a bowl.
6. Add 1 tablespoon salt plus all of the other ingredients to the warm liquid and whisk until well blended and you have a smooth sauce.
7. Pour the sauce over the beans while they are still warm and mix them up gently with a wooden spoon, being careful not to mash them.
8. Refrigerate for several hours.
9. Before serving, stir the salad again so that all the beans are well coated with the dressing.

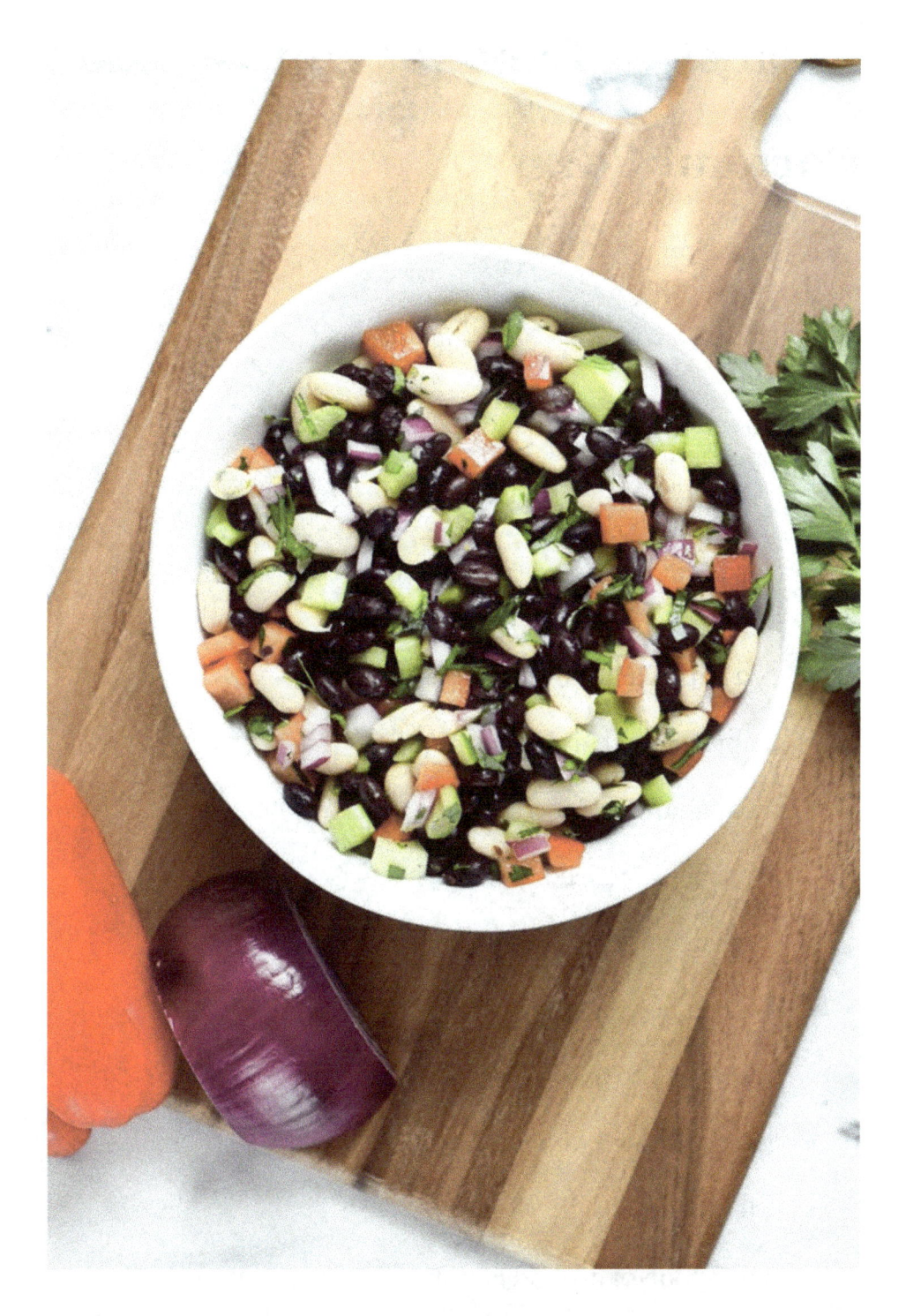

Exquisite Banana, Apple, and Coconut Curry

Servings: 6

Preparation time: 6 hours and 10 minutes

Ingredients:

- 1/2 cup of amaranth seeds
- 1 apple, cored and sliced
- 1 banana, sliced
- 1 1/2 cups of diced tomatoes
- 3 teaspoons of chopped parsley
- 1 green pepper, chopped
- 1 large white onion, peeled and diced
- 2 teaspoons of minced garlic
- 1 teaspoon of salt
- 1 teaspoon of ground cumin

- 2 1/2 tablespoons of curry powder
- 2 tablespoons of flour
- 2 bay leaves
- 1/2 cup of white wine
- 8 fluid ounce of coconut milk
- 1/2 cup of water

Directions:

1. Using a food processor place the apple, tomatoes, garlic and pulse it until it gets smooth but a little bit chunky.
2. Add this mixture to a 6-quarts slow cooker and add the remaining ingredients.
3. Stir until it mixes properly and cover the top.
4. Plug in the slow cooker; adjust the cooking time to 6 hours and let it cook on the low heat setting or until it is cooked thoroughly.
5. Add the seasoning and serve right away.

Delightful Coconut Vegetarian Curry

Servings: 6

Preparation time: 4 hours and 20 minutes

Ingredients:

- 5 medium-sized potatoes, peeled and cut into 1-inch cubes
- 1/4 cup of curry powder
- 2 tablespoons of flour
- 1 tablespoon of chili powder
- 1/2 teaspoon of red pepper flakes
- 1/2 teaspoon of cayenne pepper
- 1 large green bell pepper, cut into strips
- 1 large red bell pepper, cut into strips
- 2 tablespoons of onion soup mix

- 14-ounce of coconut cream, unsweetened
- 3 cups of vegetable broth
- 2 medium-sized carrots, peeled and cut into matchstick
- 1 cup of green peas
- 1/4 cup of chopped cilantro

Directions:

1. Take a 6-quarts slow cooker, grease it with a non-stick cooking spray and place the potatoes pieces in the bottom.
2. Add the remaining ingredients except for the carrots, peas and cilantro.
3. Stir properly and cover the top.
4. Plug in the slow cooker; adjust the cooking time to 4 hours and let it cook on the low heat setting or until it cooks thoroughly.
5. When the cooking time is over, add the carrots to the curry and continue cooking for 30 minutes.

6. Then, add the peas and continue cooking for another 30 minutes or until the peas get tender.
7. Garnish it with cilantro and serve.

Creamy Sweet Potato & Coconut Curry

Servings: 6

Preparation time: 6 hours and 20 minutes

Ingredients:

- 2 pounds of sweet potatoes, peeled and chopped
- 1/2 pound of red cabbage, shredded
- 2 red chilies, seeded and sliced
- 2 medium-sized red bell peppers, cored and sliced
- 2 large white onions, peeled and sliced
- 1 1/2 teaspoon of minced garlic

- 1 teaspoon of grated ginger
- 1/2 teaspoon of salt
- 1 teaspoon of paprika
- 1/2 teaspoon of cayenne pepper
- 2 tablespoons of peanut butter
- 4 tablespoons of olive oil
- 12-ounce of tomato puree
- 14 fluid ounce of coconut milk
- 1/2 cup of chopped coriander

Directions:

1. Place a large non-stick skillet pan over an average heat, add 1 tablespoon of oil and let it heat.
2. Then add the onion and cook for 10 minutes or until it gets soft.
3. Add the garlic, ginger, salt, paprika, cayenne pepper and continue cooking for 2 minutes or until it starts producing fragrance.
4. Transfer this mixture to a 6-quarts slow cooker, and reserve the pan.

5. In the pan, add 1 tablespoon of oil and let it heat.
6. Add the cabbage, red chili, bell pepper and cook it for 5 minutes.
7. Then transfer this mixture to the slow cooker and reserve the pan.
8. Add the remaining oil to the pan; the sweet potatoes in a single layer and cook it in 3 batches for 5 minutes or until it starts getting brown.
9. Add the sweet potatoes to the slow cooker, along with tomato puree, coconut milk and stir properly.
10. Cover the top, plug in the slow cooker; adjust the cooking time to 6 hours and let it cook on the low heat setting or until the sweet potatoes are tender.
11. When done, add the seasoning and pour it in the peanut butter.
12. Garnish it with coriander and serve.

Chives Fennel Salsa

Preparation time: 10 minutes

Cooking time: 0 minutes

Servings: 4

Ingredients:

- 2 fennel bulbs, shredded
- ½ cup chives, chopped
- Juice of 1 lime
- 2 tablespoons olive oil
- 1 cup black olives, pitted and sliced
- Salt and black pepper to the taste
- 2 celery stalks, finely chopped
- 2 tomatoes, cubed

Directions:

1. In a bowl, combine the fennel with the chives, lime juice and the other ingredients, toss well, divide into smaller bowls and serve as an appetizer.

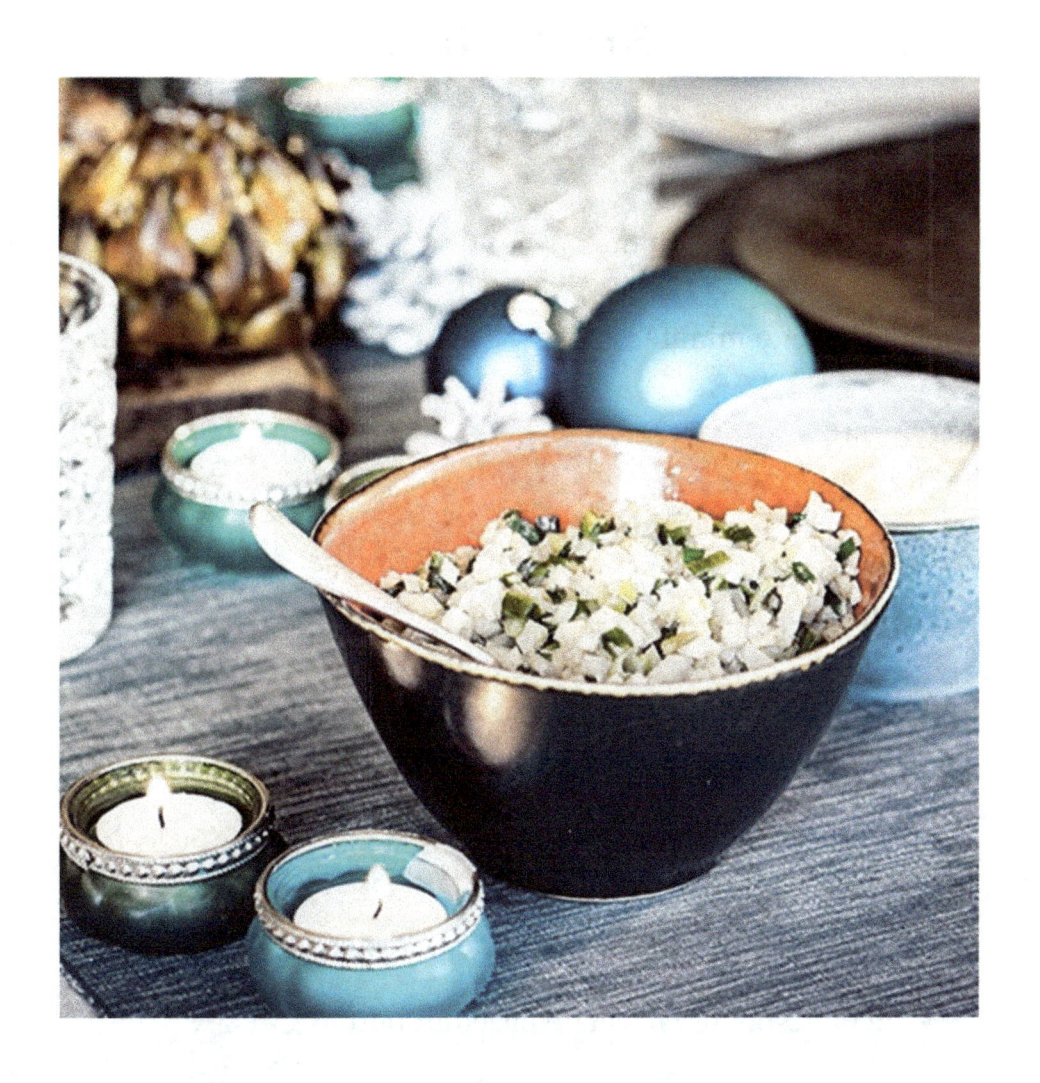

Blueberry, Hazelnut and Hemp Smoothie

Preparation time: 5 minutes

Cooking time: 0 minute

Servings: 2

Ingredients:

- 2 tablespoons hemp seeds
- 1 ½ cups frozen blueberries
- 2 tablespoons chocolate protein powder
- 1/2 teaspoon vanilla extract, unsweetened
- 2 tablespoons chocolate hazelnut butter
- 1 small frozen banana
- 3/4 cup almond milk

Directions:

1. Place all the ingredients in the order in a food processor or blender and then pulse for 2 to 3 minutes at high speed until smooth.
2. Pour the smoothie into two glasses and then serve.

Mocha Chocolate Shake

Preparation time: 5 minutes

Cooking time: 0 minute

Servings: 2

Ingredients:

- 1/4 cup hemp seeds
- 2 teaspoons cocoa powder, unsweetened
- 1/2 cup dates, pitted
- 1 tablespoon instant coffee powder
- 2 tablespoons flax seeds
- 2 1/2 cups almond milk, unsweetened
- 1/2 cup crushed ice

Directions:

1. Place all the ingredients in the order in a food processor or blender and then pulse for 2 to 3 minutes at high speed until smooth.
2. Pour the smoothie into two glasses and then serve.

96

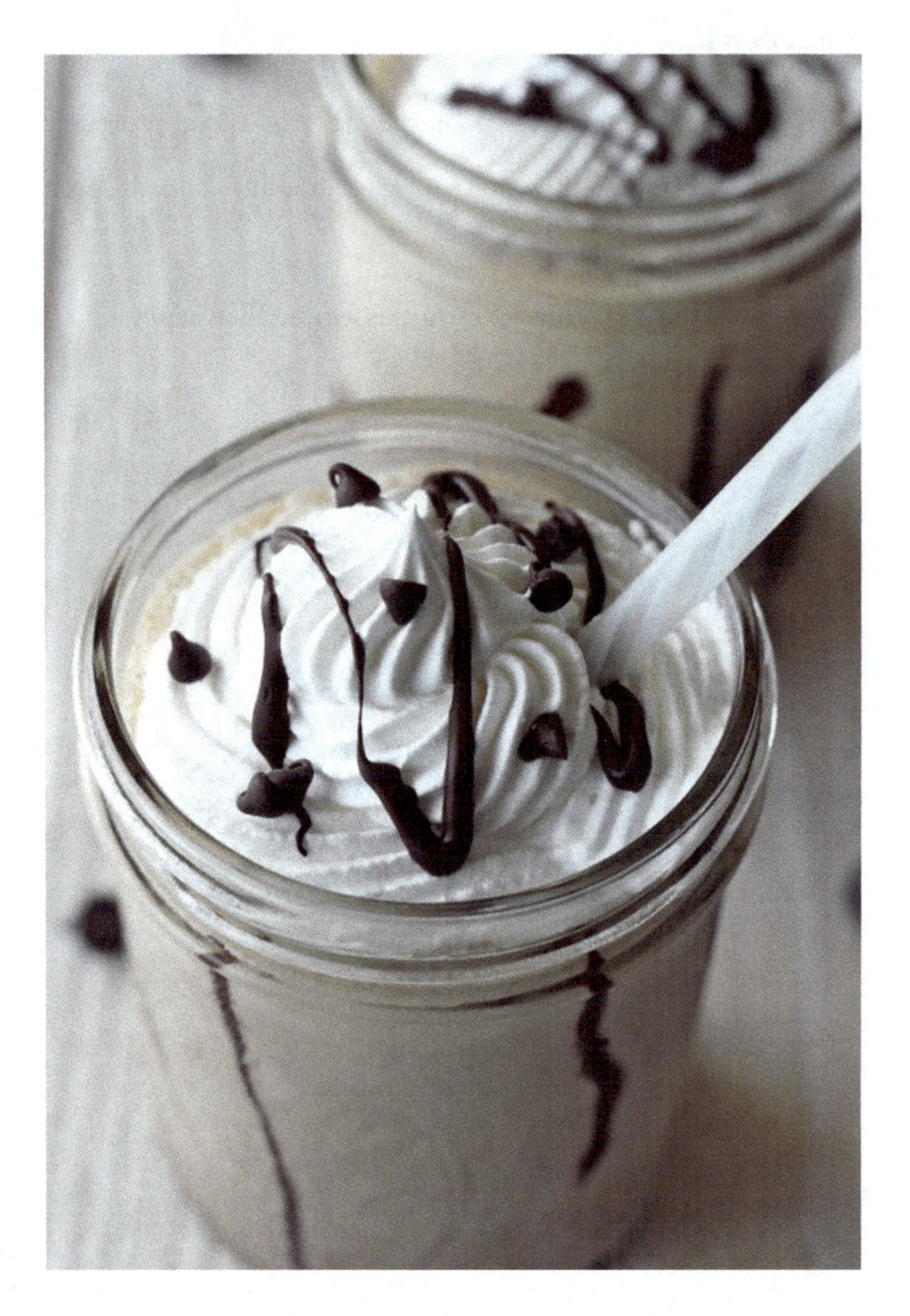

Red Beet, Pear and Apple Smoothie

Preparation time: 5 minutes

Cooking time: 0 minute

Servings: 2

Ingredients:

- 1/2 of medium beet, peeled, chopped
- 1 tablespoon chopped cilantro
- 1 orange, juiced
- 1 medium pear, chopped
- 1 medium apple, cored, chopped
- 1/4 teaspoon ground black pepper
- 1/8 teaspoon rock salt
- 1 teaspoon coconut sugar

- 1/4 teaspoons salt
- 1 cup of water

Directions:

1. Place all the ingredients in the order in a food processor or blender and then pulse for 2 to 3 minutes at high speed until smooth.
2. Pour the smoothie into two glasses and then serve.

Chocolate and Cherry Smoothie

Preparation time: 5 minutes

Cooking time: 0 minute

Servings: 2

Ingredients:

- 4 cups frozen cherries
- 2 tablespoons cocoa powder
- 1 scoop of protein powder
- 1 teaspoon maple syrup
- 2 cups almond milk, unsweetened

Directions:

1. Place all the ingredients in the order in a food processor or blender and then pulse for 2 to 3 minutes at high speed until smooth.
2. Pour the smoothie into two glasses and then serve.

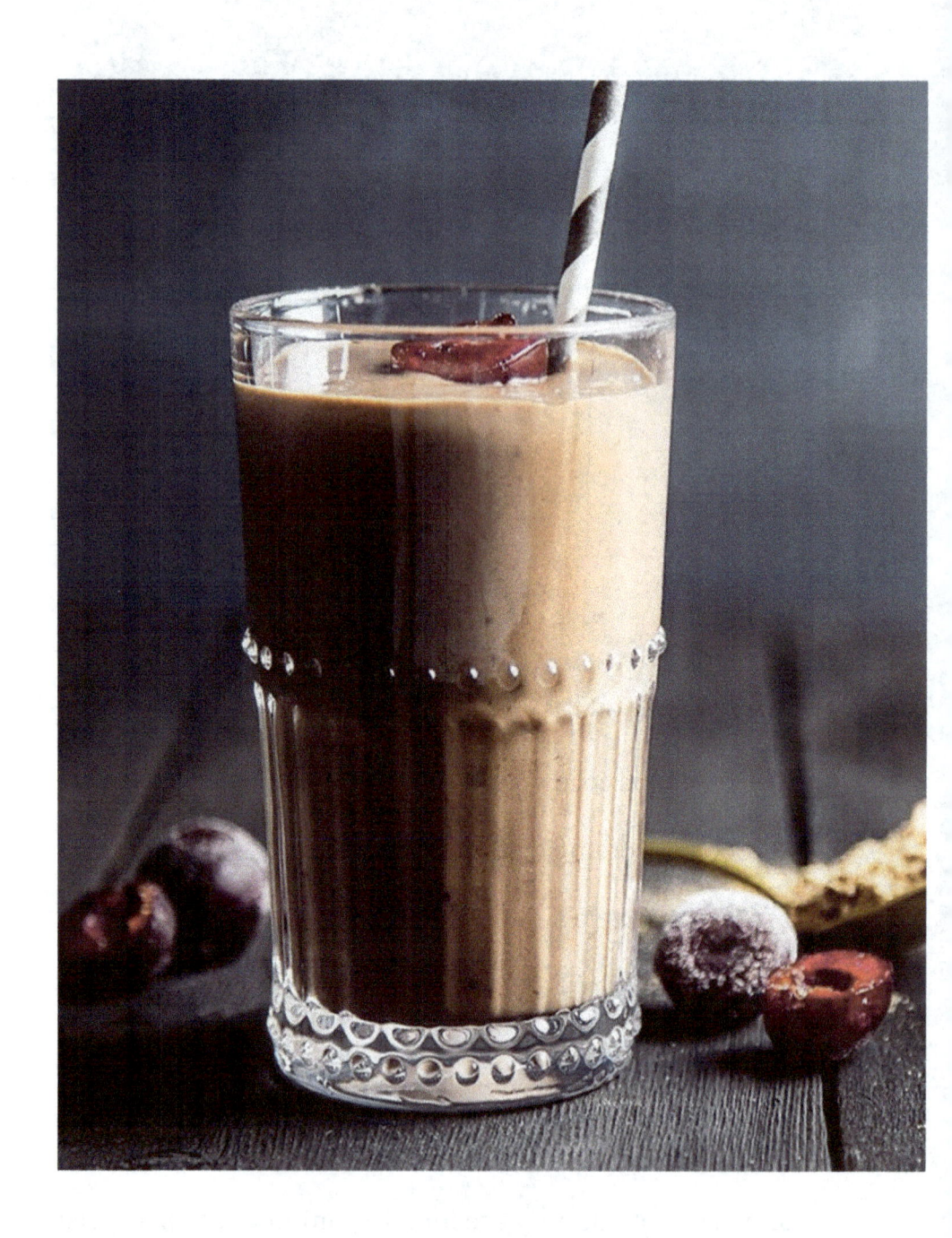

Banana and Protein Smoothie

Preparation time: 5 minutes

Cooking time: 0 minute

Servings: 2

Ingredients:

- 2/3 cup frozen pineapple chunk
- 10 frozen strawberries
- 2 frozen bananas
- 2 scoops protein powder
- 2 teaspoons cocoa powder
- 2 tablespoons maple syrup
- 2 teaspoons vanilla extract, unsweetened
- 2 cups almond milk, unsweetened

Directions:

1. Place all the ingredients in the order in a food processor or blender and then pulse for 2 to 3 minutes at high speed until smooth.
2. Pour the smoothie into two glasses and then serve.

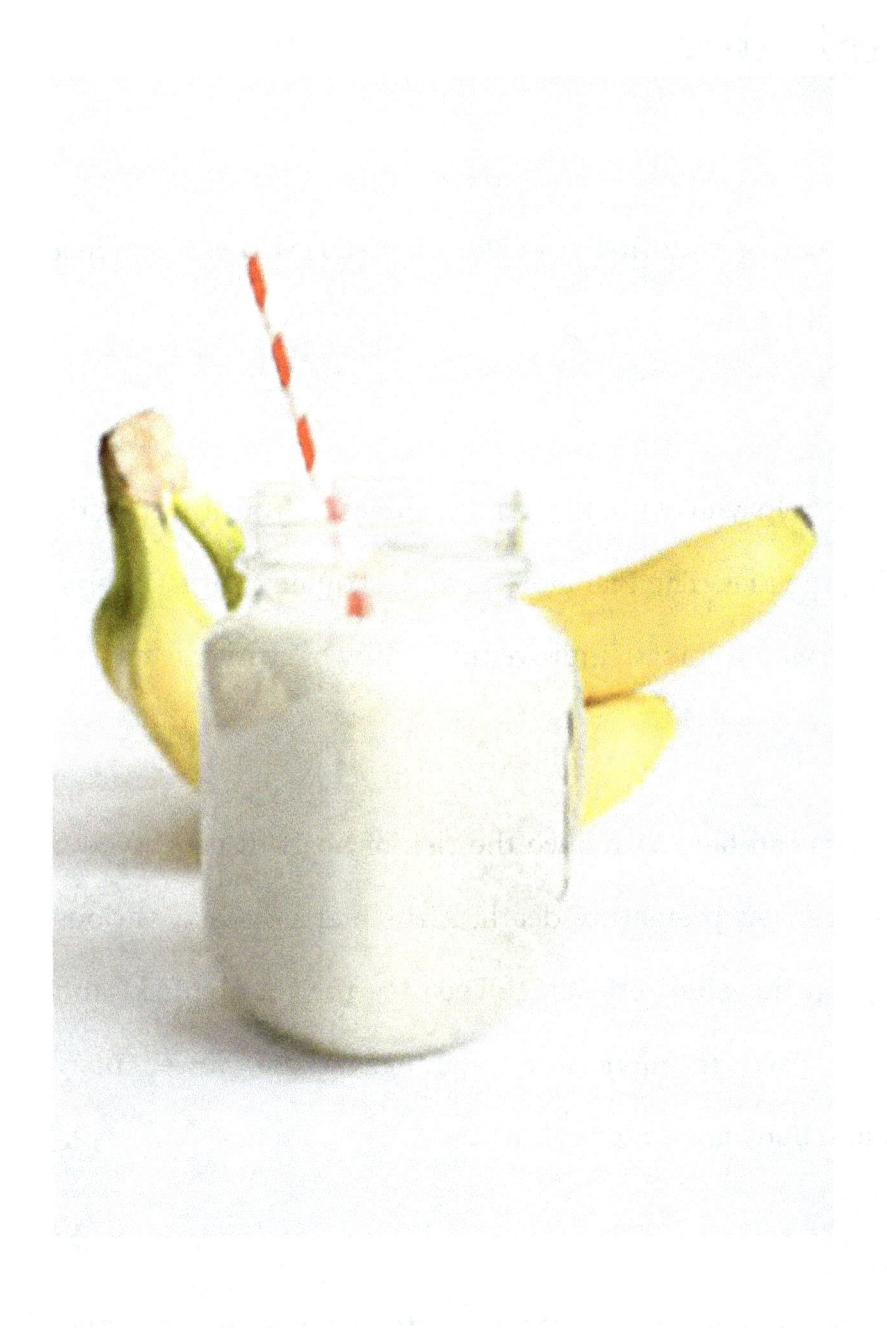

Conclusion

This book can be your first guide for Plant-Based Diet if you just started your journey.

Or it can help you with the recipe choice if you are already following the diet. The Plant-Based and Alkaline diet is suitable for anyone who wants to improve the quality of everyday life.

These diets can help to reduce the risk of heart disease, type 2 diabetes, cancer, premature death, Alzheimer's disease, various cancers, avoid side effects linked to the antibiotics and hormones used in modern animal agriculture, lower body weight and body mass index (BMI).

Usually, people decide to go vegan due to one or several reasons. People might switch to veganism due to their ethical reasons, as they believe all live creatures have a right to live, be free, and fairly treated.

You can find your reasons. There are many sources of healthy nutrients in vegan products. So you don't have to worry about getting enough vitamins to your body.

This book will help you to make a healthy vegan Meal Plan for the whole family and spend less time in the kitchen. Remember that Veganism is not only about the diet, but about changing your lifestyle to a more healthy and balanced one. And this book will help you with this.

You can choose the recipe you like from a variety of options: Breakfast recipes Bread and Biscuits Salads and Soups Main dishes Smoothies and Teas Sauces and condiments Desserts Snacks Whole Food recipes

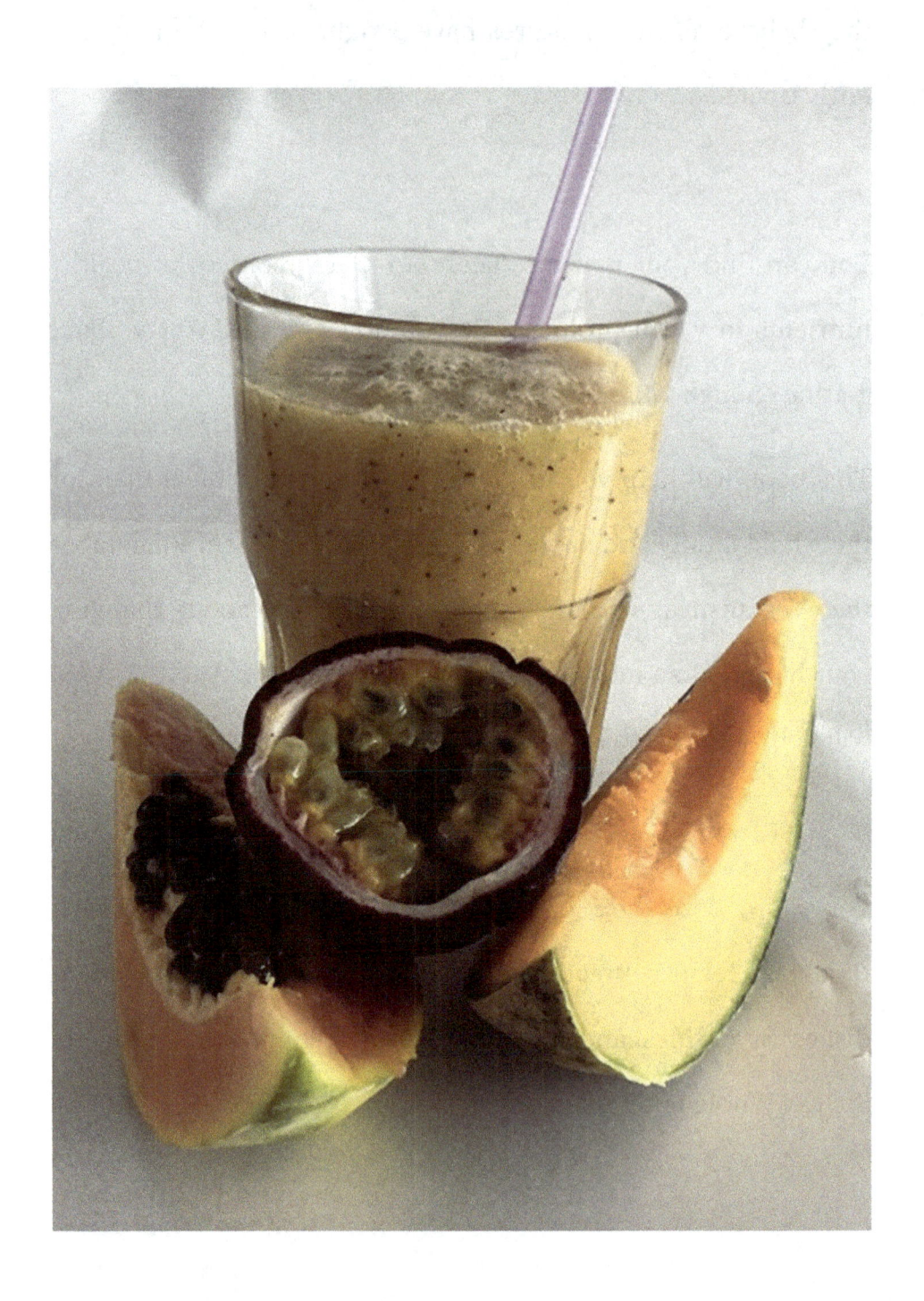